MW00928870

YOGA FOR ABSOLUTE BEGINNERS

YOGA

FOR **ABSOLUTE**
BEGINNERS

*Poses for Relaxation, Stress Reduction,
Weight Loss, Improved Flexibility and
Muscle Strength*

Oliver Crawford

Table of Contents

Preface

This book was designed for those who have no prior experience of doing yoga. The postures included in this book are aimed at the absolute beginners. Apart from the clear instruction for each posture, yoga breathing or pranayama techniques were applied to each exercise so that the benefits are multiplied. Asanas (Postures) were designed maintaining Astanga Vinyasa (Sequential yoga postures combined with Hatha yoga and Pranayama). It is advised to do the advanced poses in the presence of an expert yoga practitioner, although most of the postures included in this book can be practiced without help or supervision. If you have musculoskeletal pain, neck injury; consult your doctor before practicing. Many of the poses are not suitable during pregnancy. Therefore, it is recommended to consult a physician before starting yoga exercises. Yoga has become popular for countless health benefits and practitioners will start to experience positive changes within a couple of weeks after starting Yoga. This book, however, was not written as a treatment alternative for those who are already receiving medical treatment or in a need for medical attention.

Chapter 1

A brief introduction to Yoga

Yoga for its numerous health benefits has become a part of life for millions across the globe. Anyone can practice Yoga, it does not require instruments, and it does not have any age restriction. General physical exercises focus on physical well-being, and Yoga focuses on balancing, by ensuring a sound body as well as a sound mind. The word Yoga derived from its Sanskrit root "Yog" which means union. Practicing yoga creates a union between the body and the mind, between the body-mind and nature. And when the union is created, an amazing balancing takes place. For the last several decades, potentials of yoga for healing diseases have become a topic of research. Yoga has become an effective alternative treatment approach for various physical and psychological ailments. Yoga does not just cures diseases; it prolongs the lifespan, that's why the word 'rejuvenation' is often uttered as an attribute to yoga. Although it's popularly known as a physical exercise, yoga has many other aspects. As a matter of fact, physical exercise covers a tiny part of the vast Yogic scriptures. But since our aim is to use yoga as a practice for improving our physical and psychological state, we will discuss two aspects of Yoga. One is Hatha yoga; a physical exercise consisted of thousands of postures (Asanas and Mudras), and the other is Pranayama, yogic breathing exercise.

Among the thousands of yoga postures, some postures are basic, can be practiced with ease, some are intermediate which requires some degrees of strength and flexibility following a little caution, and some are advanced which requires some level of physical fitness and supervision in the beginning. Therefore there are few one-size-fits-all postures. However, we don't need to learn all of them, learning ten to twelve postures are more than enough. In this book, we will start from the very basic yoga postures and move towards more advanced level by gradually adding features. Some postures may look difficult at the beginning, but with few days practice, the flexibility and endurance will improve. Yoga can be practiced at any time of the day. But the ideal time is morning, on an empty stomach or 3-4 hours after a large meal. Ideal duration is between 15 to 90 minutes. But even a few minutes of regular practice will make a difference. Some of the poses are specialised, targeting certain groups, aimed at strengthening certain parts of the body or eliminating certain physical or mental illnesses and some are age restricted. A little warm up is recommended before trying strenuous postures. Warm up postures may include twisting, forward and backward bend, sun salutation is also a good warm up if someone is comfortable with it.

Getting prepared

Yoga has to be practiced on bare feet. Clothing should be loose but not too loose, cotton tight and t-shirt is ok. Do not push yourself beyond your limit; there is no competition here and no struggling. But regularity and persistence is paramount for gaining the mastery. If you feel hungry, eat some light snacks and wait for a while; if thirsty, drink some water. Find a quiet place where you won't be disturbed, turn off your TV, cell phone but a soothing music is ok. If you are practicing outside your home, avoid crowded places and direct sunlight. Although no instrument is necessary, you can use some (i.e. yoga block, yoga ball) if you like. If you are practicing on a highly polished floor, use a mat (ideally yoga mat) to avoid slipping and sliding. Remember to breathe, and don't hold your breath while doing yoga. There are instructions for inhaling and exhaling during movements; we will learn it as we move on.

Chapter 2

Attaining Flexibility

The flexibility of human body is closely related to longevity. Our body grows rigid, as we grow older; when flexibility improves, it slows down aging. Yoga counteracts aging in many ways; developing flexibility is one of them. The extent of flexibility determines the level of physical fitness. A flexible body has a lower risk of injury. While we boost our flexibility doing yoga postures by stretching different muscle groups, it also improves blood circulation. Better blood circulation promotes the body's immunity and cut the risks of various diseases. In this chapter, we will start with very simple and easy yoga postures for attaining physical flexibility.

Warming up

Sit in a comfortable position placing your palms on your knees, with your spine straight. Feel as comfortable as you can. Allow the lower part of your body to completely rest on the floor. Feel relaxed and keep your head straight. Take a long deep breath and exhale slowly.

Now gently rotate your head to the right while breathing in. Rotate your head to the left while breathing out. Again, to the right, breathe in and to the left, breathe out. Do it four times. Lower your chin toward your chest and hold the position for five seconds.

Lower your right ear towards your left shoulder while keeping the spine straight, and hold the contraction for five seconds. Take your left ear toward your left shoulder and hold for five seconds.

Slowly stand up with your legs apart. Stand firmly and make sure your weight is evenly distributed on both legs. Inhale and lift your arms up with palms facing each other. Exhale and lower your arms. Again inhale and raise your arms, exhale and lower your arms. Do it at least four times.

Raise your arms up to the shoulder level, inhale and rotate your torso to the right, keep the hand and shoulder straight. Exhale and rotate your torso to the right. Again, breathe in and twist to the right, breathe out and twist to the left.

Inhale and bend your body forward, exhale and bend your body backward. One more round, inhale, bend forward; exhale, bend backward.

Now, breathe in, bend your body to the right. Breathe out; bend your body to the left. Do it one more time.

The following poses were designed maintaining Astanga vinyasa, sequential yoga postures combined with hatha yoga and pranayama.

Mountain Pose (Tadasana)

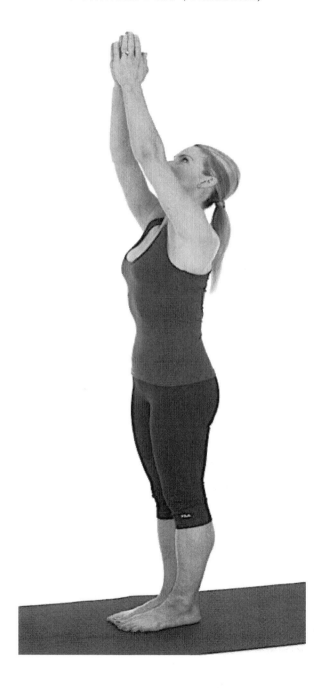

Tadasana

Stand with you heels slightly apart. Stand straight and make sure your weight is evenly distributed on both feet, and your chin parallel to the floor. Correct your position by slightly moving your head to align with the centre of your pelvis. Now, breathe in and lift your chin, raise your hands from the sides with palms facing each other. Join your palms together and stretch your arms and reach your fingers towards the sky. Push your pelvis slightly forward, and breathe naturally. Stay in this position for 30 seconds. Switch to the next pose once you're done.

Benefits: Heals back pain, strengthens legs, improves focus.

Warrior Pose 1 (Virabhadrasana-1)

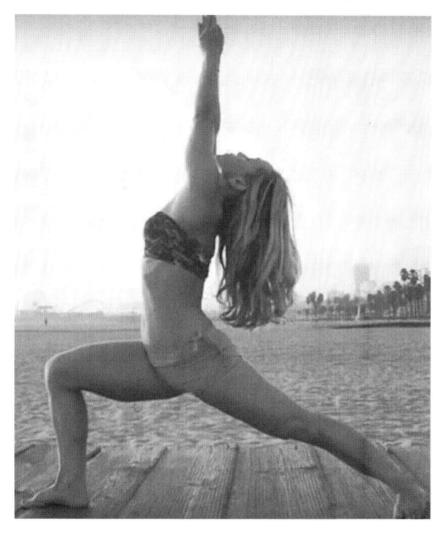

Warrior pose-1

If you are using a mat, step back your left leg. And position it parallel to the width and your right leg 45 degrees to the length of the mat. Align the position of your heels. Bend your right knee and if possible, place your sheen perpendicular and your thigh parallel to the floor. You don't have to be perfect in this at the beginning, so stretch as much as you can. Lift your both arms and join the palms together (as described in mountain pose). Breathe normally and stay in this position for a while. Change the position of your legs. This time, step back your right leg and bend your left knee, squeeze your palms together and breathe naturally.

Benefits: This pose is great for cardiac health. Warrior pose-1 improves blood circulation in lungs and heart. It strengthens the muscles in chest, belly, back, shoulders, arms and legs.

Warrior Pose 2 (Virabhadrasana-2)

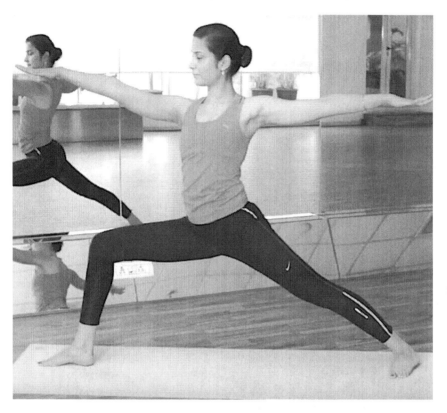

Warrior pose-2

Warrior pose two is different from pose one in terms of the position of the hands. Move your left leg backward and bend your right knee as described in pose-1. Stretch your arms parallel to the floor and rest your gaze on the top of the right middle finger. Remain in this position for 30 seconds to a minute. Change your leg, and this time, bend your left knee and practice for 30 seconds.

Benefits: Warrior pose-2 is beneficial to the circulatory and respiratory system. Apart from strengthening the limbs, it energises the whole body.

Tree Pose (Vrikshasana)

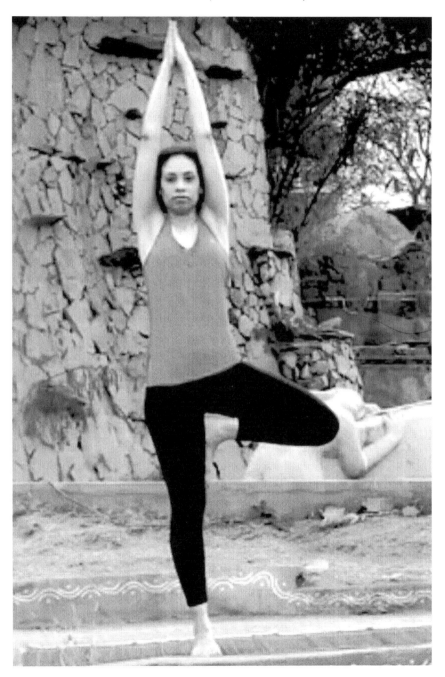

Tree Pose

Stand firm on the ground with feet slightly apart. Bend your right knee and rest your right heel against the left inner-thigh. Breathe in and lift your hand from sides with palms facing each other. Squeeze your palms together and breathe normally. Breathe 10-15 times, and then gently lower right leg and hands. Repeat on the other side. If you are having difficulty balancing your body while putting your weight on one leg, you can practice it close to the wall in the beginning. If you are comfortable with this posture, you can improvise a little by bending to the right and left a few times.

Benefits: Tree pose increases the balancing of the body. It also firms the leg muscles and increases memory, concentration and focus.

Downward-facing dog (Adho-Mukha Svanasana)

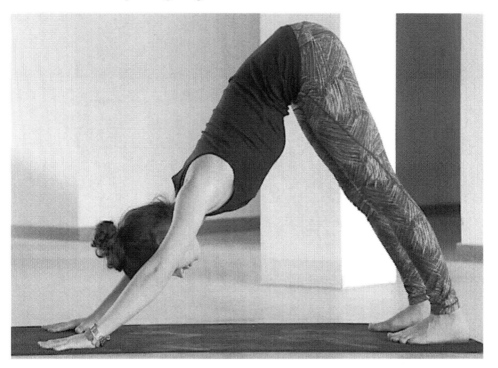

Downward-facing dog

This pose will relax your thighs after you've finished the above positions. Sit on your ankles. Bend your torso from the waist and rest on your thighs. Straighten your hands and place your palms on the floors around 20 cm apart with fingers spread, inhale. Exhale, raise your torso and put your weight on your hands and knees, inhale. Exhale and lift your knees off the floor and straighten your legs. Face downward and legs slightly apart; inhale and breathe normally for 10 to 100 times. Beginners can use a yoga block to support the head during this pose.

Benefits: This pose increases the blood circulation of the body, releases stress, anxiety and boosts energy.

Corpse pose (Savasana)

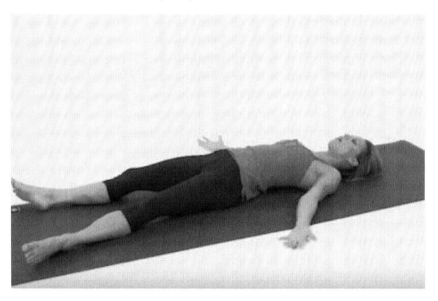

Savasana

Traditionally this pose is practiced at the end, but you can also practice in the beginning to calm your mind. Therefore if you want to end your practice for today, you can use this posture. Otherwise move to the next chapter, try some other poses and once you are done, practice Savasana. Here are the steps you have to follow. Lie comfortably on your back with you hand by your side slightly apart, palms facing the ceiling, legs apart. Close your eyes. Take a slow deep breath and exhale slowly, spend more time on out-breathing. Do it a couple more rounds. Now breathe naturally, let your body sink into the floor. Pay your attention from head to toe. Let your head relax with every in-breath. Imagine all your tension is leaving the body with each exhale. Focus on your neck, your chest, your back, your hand, your belly your hips your thighs, knees, sheens, calves, ankles, feet; spend five seconds on each part, breathe normally. Relax your body with each breath; pay your attention to your breath. Stay in this position for ten minutes.

Benefits: Savasana releases stress and anxiety, improves focus, stills the mind, normalises cardiovascular activities and on the top, it gives you a proper rest.

Chapter 3

Stronger muscles and perfect weight

Yoga offers tremendous benefits for your musculoskeletal health by strengthening muscle tone and improving blood circulation in the muscles of your body. In this chapter, we will be practicing some little advanced poses. Yoga postures included in this chapter is aimed at improving muscle tone, joint strength, and firmness of abs muscles. Those who want to lose weight and attain a perfect, well-balanced figure will find the following asanas very effective.

Prior to practicing these postures, do some warm-up poses described in the previous chapter.

Triangle Pose (Trikonasana)

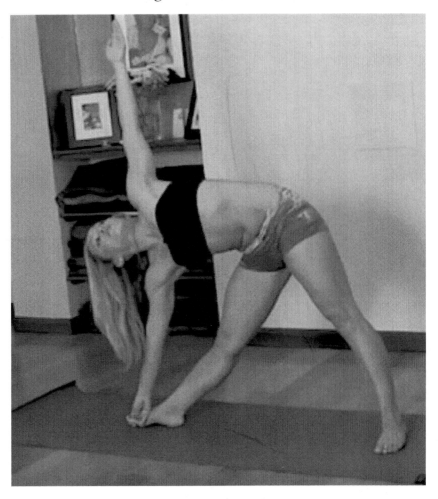

Trikonasana

Stand firmly on the ground and step your feet wide apart. Position your feet as described in warrior pose. You can switch directly from warrior pose to triangle pose if you want. But this time, don't bend your knees instead, straighten your legs. Now, your right foot is positioned forward and left foot is positioned backward. Lower your right hand and touch the ground next to your heel or hold your big toe (both positions are correct). Stretch your left hand toward the ceiling. Make sure your hands are aligned to your shoulder and perpendicular to the floor. Fix your gaze on the tip of middle finger of your left hand. Breathe in and breathe out in this position for few times. Depending on the flexibility of your body, you may need a yoga block to support your hand on the ground, but it is optional; bend as much as you can; don't try harder. If you are having difficulty with balancing, do this posture against the wall. After you've finished with the right side, change the position of your leg and try it on the left side following the instructions.

Benefits: This pose strengthens the joints in your hands and legs. It also firms the muscles in abdomen and thorax. Triangle pose is also beneficial for improving digestion and relieving stress.

Caution: Avoid this asana if you have back pain, insomnia, and low blood pressure. Also, avoid this asana if you are pregnant.

Plank Pose (Phalakasana)

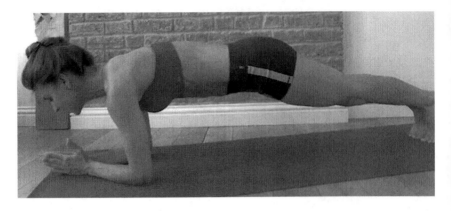

Phalakasana

You can switch to this position from the downward facing dog (Adho Mukha Svanasana). Otherwise, start with Adhamukha Svanasana, and lower your torso and make sure your arms are perpendicular and thorax is parallel to the floor; straighten your body (plank – position). Shift your gaze at the floor. Breathe in and breathe out at least five times while staying in this asana. Once finished, bend and shift your weight on your knees. Sit on your ankle and get your hands off the floor.

Benefits: Plank pose strengthens your wrists, shoulders and improves the muscle tone in your chest and abdomen. This posture cuts the risks of back pain.

Child Pose (Balasana)

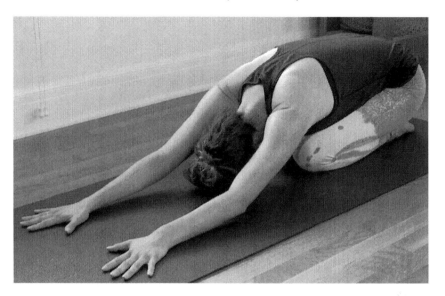

Balasana

Child pose is a relaxing posture. You can switch to child pose from plank pose safely. Or you can use this pose as a preparatory position for the next pose. Sit on your ankles, and bend your torso from your waist. Straighten your hands and rest your forehead on the ground. Touch the floor with your both palms slightly apart in a resting position (it is alright if your elbows touch the ground). You can also place your hands by your side with palms facing upward (choose either of the hand positions). Breathe in and out in this posture for at least 30 seconds. Child pose is supposed to be a very relaxing posture, although some of you may find it little difficult in the beginning. It is important to pay attention while doing this posture. Don't let your mind drift away; you can either focus on your breath or your forehead.

Benefits: Child pose calms the mind and releases anxiety and anger. This pose also relieves the practitioner from fatigue and dizziness. It also relieves back pain.

Thunderbolt Pose (Vajrasana)

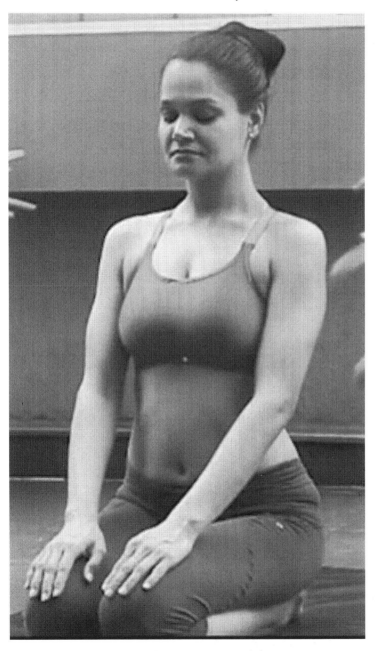

Vajrasana

Sit on your heels, make sure the soles of your feet are positioned either side of your anus and your knees and feet are slightly apart. Your thighs will rest on your calves with your hands resting on your thighs. Keep your spine and head straight. Look straight or close your eyes. If you are having difficulty sitting like this, you can use a folded blanket to sit on. Breathe normally and focus. This pose can be practiced as a part of your yoga practice or immediately after a heavy meal (lunch and dinner) to accelerate digestion. If you are practicing after a meal, try to stay in this position for at least fifteen minutes and drink a glass of water afterwards.

Benefits: This asana is good for both dyspepsia and constipation. Vajrasana accelerates blood flow in the digestive system and hence improves the digestion. Vajrasana also firms the abdomen and increases confidence. People with irritable bowel syndrome (IBS) will find this position particularly beneficial. Practice Vajrasana if you want strong abdomen and stronger confidence.

More advanced positions

The following two positions are for the advanced practitioners. But the beginners with a flexible body can practice it too. If you are comfortable with Halasana, also try Chakrasana, as they are sequential poses.

Plough Pose (Halasana)

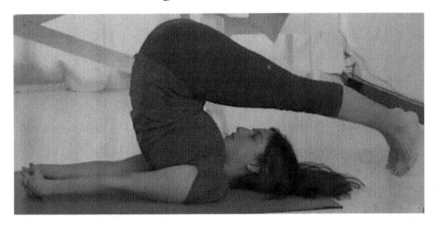

Halasana

Lie down on your back with hands by your side and your palms touching the floor. Breathe in; breath out and lift your legs off the ground; to support the lifting, put pressure on your hands; lower your feet toward your forehead and rest them on the floor. Keep your legs straight and bring your hands together (behind your back) with palms facing each other. Lock the fingers together. Your torso should be perpendicular to the floor, and your chin is slightly apart from your sternum. It is better if you can make some room between your chin and sternum to relax your throat. You can use a folded blanket to support your head and hands. If you find it difficult to lower your legs, you can use a yoga block, even a chair if the block is too low. Remember to breathe in and out. The ideal duration for this position is between one and five minutes. Locking your fingers is not mandatory; you can rest your palms on the floor if you are practicing it for the first time.

Benefits: There are numerous benefits of Halasana including firming abdominal muscles, reducing fat, relieving stress. Diabetic people will find this pose very helpful. Halasana also reduces the symptoms of menopause. This position counteracts aging. If you want a beautiful glowing skin, practice Halasana.

Caution: This is an advanced posture. If you are practicing for the first time and not feeling confident enough, try it under the supervision of an expert practitioner. Halasana is not for everyone; this pose requires some degree of physical flexibility.

Wheel Pose (Chakrasana)

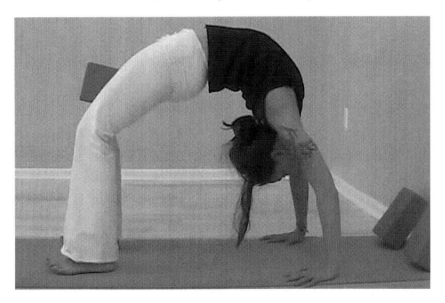

Chakrasana

In Sanskrit, Chakra means wheel; therefore this posture is supposed to look like a wheel or semi-wheel. Lie on your back, breathe in and exhale. Bend your knees and rest your feet on the floor 15 cm apart. Bend your elbows and rest your palms on either side of your head aligning your shoulders, and fingers spread. Place your feet away from your buttocks, so that your calves are slightly away from your thighs. Breathe in; breathe out and lift your torso by pressing your feet and palms. Try to straighten your hands and legs so that your spine is pushed up and form a circular shape. Remember to inhale and exhale and hold the position between 15 to 30 seconds.

Benefits: Chakrasana improves vitality. Strengthens ankles and grips and firms the muscles of hands, legs and torso. This pose improves balancing and flexibility. Good for sexual health. Like Halasana, Chakrasana also counteracts aging.

Caution: To avoid sliding your palms and feet during posture, do not use too smooth surface. A yoga mat is better if you are practicing indoor. As this is an advanced pose, it is advisable for beginners to practice this asana under the supervision of an expert practitioner. But if you are confident and have a flexible body, go ahead.

Chapter 4

Living a longer life

Physical exercises, in general, are practiced for staying physically fit and maintaining a healthy living. General physical exercises offer health benefits. Yoga not only offers good health, but it also offers longevity. There are tons of examples of people who managed to lower the process of aging, using the powerful yoga techniques, and thriving at the age of ninety. Our genetic predisposition has a lot to contribute to our lifespan. However, adopting yoga as a part of life will slow down the aging process. But in order to get the most out of anti-aging yoga, we have to follow some fundamental rules of healthy living. The rules are as follows.

One: Eating balanced diets in a timely manner,

Two: Drinking plenty of water

Three: Having a proper sleep (At least eight hours a day)

Four: Include lots of fruits and vegetables in diets.

Most of the yoga postures contribute to anti-aging. But the asanas we are about to discuss in this chapter are more effective when it comes to gaining rejuvenation and vitality. We will practice eleven postures in this chapter. You are already familiar with few of them. When those postures are practiced sequentially, the process is called Sun Salutation or Surya Namaskar. But before learning Sun Salutation, let us learn the elements of this posture, or the asanas, which were not covered in the previous chapters.

Prayer Pose (Pranamasa)

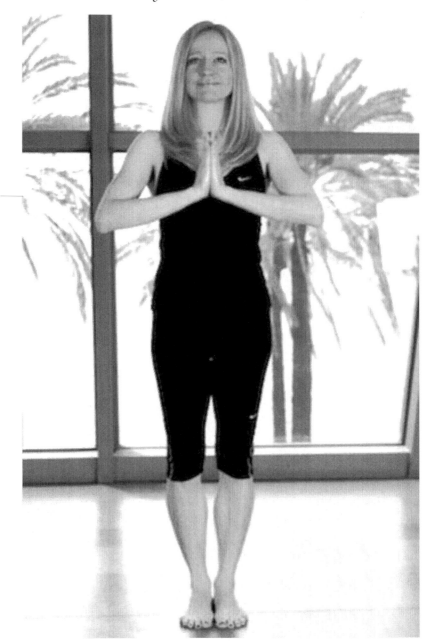

Pranamasana

Stand at the edge of your mat with feet slightly apart. Straighten your torso and make sure that both of your feet are equally carrying your weight. Feel that your feet are planted firmly on the floor, and your body is growing upward from your feet to the tip of your head. Head straight… Gaze straight. Breathe in and bend your arms from the elbow and clasp the palms together before your chest. Breath out, and slightly stretch your forearms to make sure that they are parallel to the floor. Relax your shoulders and feel your chest opening up. Breathe out and feel the pressure between your palms. Breathe normally and stay in this position for thirty seconds.

Visualisation: You can close your eyes during this posture and rest your attention on the Anahata Chakra or the heart Chakra. Bring the feeling of positivity, feel the nourishing energy in your heart chakra, breathe normally and stay with this energy.

Benefits: Pranamasana improves the sense of balance, promotes vitality, strengthens the neck muscles and makes us mentally strong.

Hand to Feet Pose (Hasta Padasana)

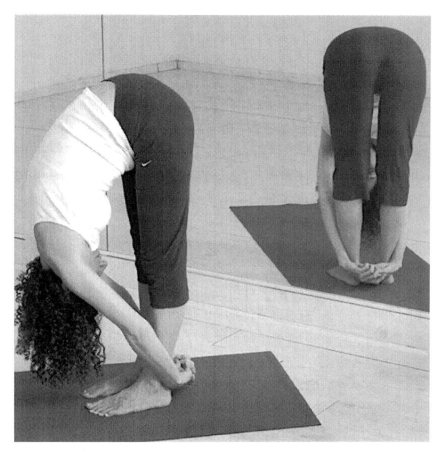

Hasta Padasana 1

This posture looks a little advanced, but it is not. Before we start this posture, remember that you don't have to be perfect at this early stage. Perfection will come in time.

Stand erect as described in pranamasana. Breathe in and raise your hands. Breathe out and bend your body forward… keep bending until your hands touch your feet. If you find it difficult to bend that low, bend as much as you can. You can use a yoga brick (not mandatory) to rest your hands. If your hands can reach up to your ankles, grab your ankles with your hands.

If you can reach up to the toes, hold your toes. You can use another method: First bend your knees to hold your big toes. Then slowly straighten your legs. If you are flexible, your belly will eventually touch your thighs. Stretch your belly slightly toward the thighs to prevent the chest from sinking in.

Whether you can touch your feet or ankles, keep your legs straight. While you are resting in this position, feel the stress-points in your legs, your torso, your hands, and your neck…. Breathe normally and stay with the feeling. Stay in this posture for fifteen seconds.

This posture has several variations. But, since we are practicing beginners' yoga, we will use the easiest pose. It is advisable not to try too hard to reach the ideal state of this posture. Don't use drastic force to bend your body to reach your toes. Breathe deeply and stretch slowly. Bend the body as much as you can, but don't struggle. If you practice regularly, you will be better at this.

Benefits: This Asana stimulates the nervous and endocrine system, aids the blood circulation in the head, boosts digestion and rejuvenates the body.

Caution: Hasta Padasana is not recommended for people with chronic back pain, and spinal problems. If you are recovering from an injury in your hips, legs, shoulders and back, avoid doing this pose.

Equestrian pose (Ashwa Sanchalanasana)

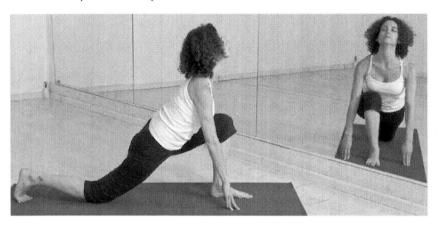

Ashwa Sanchalanasana 1

Kneel down with your knees and feet slightly apart. Bring your hands to the floor. Place your palms around 20 cm apart with fingers spread. The knees should be in alignment with the waist.

Now your hands, knees, and toes are touching the ground. Your torso is parallel to the floor. Breathe in, lift your knees and straighten your legs. Balance yourself in this position and exhale.

Inhale and step your left foot forward. Position your left foot between your palms. Push your right leg back and rest your right knee on the floor. Exhale.

Inhale and with your fingers touching the ground, lift your head and shoulder. Tilt your head back and release your breath. Breathe naturally and stay in this position for a while. Once you are done, step your left foot back and straighten your legs. Now step your right foot forward, lower your left knee and follow the same instructions.

Benefits: Equestrian pose harmonises the nervous system, gives a sense of nervous balance, improves flexibility, strengthens the spine and improves vigour.

Stick Pose (Dandasana)

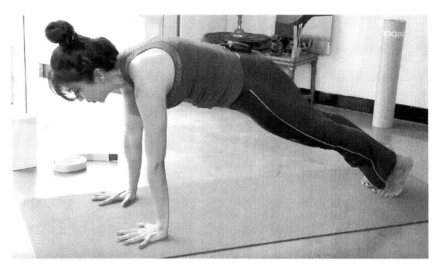

Dandasana 1

If you have already learnt the previous pose (Equestrian pose), you already know how to balance the body in Dandasana. This pose has several variations. But as we are going to practice Dandasana as a part of sun salutation, we will practice the posture the easiest way.

Kneel down as described in the previous pose. Now bring your hands to the floor. Place your palms forward, few inches from the line of shoulder. Your weight is evenly distributed on your hands and knees. Breathe deeply and exhale. Breathe again…. Exhale and get your knees off the floor and straighten your legs. You may need to push your feet back to straighten your whole body.

Breathe normally and stay in this position for thirty seconds.

Benefits: Stick pose promotes blood circulation. It is good for your cardiac health. It is also a preventative posture for back pain.

Salute With Eight Parts Or Points (Ashtanga Namaskara)

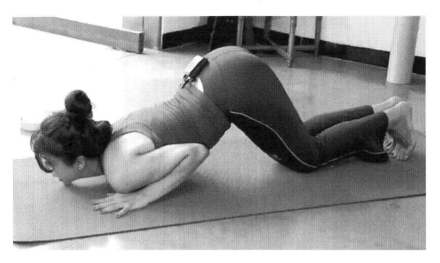

Astanga Namaskar

This Asana is also called Eight Limbed Salutation. During this posture, the body touches the floor at eight points: Two feet, two knees, two palms, the chest and the head. Sanskrit term 'Asta' means eight and 'Anga' means limb.

Sit down on your heels. Take a deep breath. Exhale and bring your body to the kneeling position. Lower your torso and touch the floor with your palms and chest. Your hands and knees will carry the most of the weight of your body. Keep pressure in your belly. Now your palms are placed on either side of your shoulder; your chin is carrying the weight of your head, or you can lightly touch the floor with your chin. Make sure there is a comfortable distance between your chin and your knees. Correct your position by pushing the knees backward. Remember to breathe in and out in this position. Stay in this asana for at least ten seconds. If you are interested in mantra, you can gently say, 'Om Pushne Namaha'. This means, 'Salutation to the one who gives strength.' Mantra is not mandatory, but some practitioners prefer to practice it in a yogic way to improve the experience. But it is important to focus on the stress points to get the most out of this posture. When you are done, push the floor with your palms to lift the torso off the ground and switch to the sitting position. Place your palms on your thighs and relax for a while.

Benefits: Astanga Namaskar strengthens the muscles of hands, legs and chest. This Asana also helps to beat depression and anxiety.

Cobra Pose (Bhujangasana)

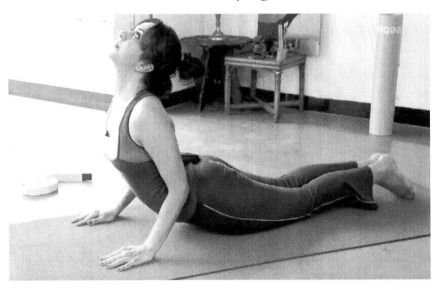

Bhujangasana

Lie down on your belly and place your palms on either side of your shoulder. Straighten you legs. To do it correctly, lift your left leg and stretch. Then roll your thigh in, lower your leg and reach the floor first with your pinky toe… then place all your toes on the floor and press gently. Raise the right leg and do the same. Now all your toes are equally touching the floor.

Breath in and with your legs touching the ground, lift your torso by straightening your hands. If you find it difficult to stretch your hands fully, leave your hands slightly bent and hold this posture. Make sure your belly is not touching the floor and your toe fingers, knees and thighs are in contact with the floor. Move your shoulders away from your ears and tilt your head back. This posture resembles a serpent with its hood raised. Breathe in and out naturally in this position. Stay for ten seconds. Once done, lower your torso, and lie on your belly.

Benefits: Cobra pose relieves back pain, invigorates the heart and elevates the mood. It is a good stretch for the muscles in abdomen and buttocks.

Caution: Although cobra pose prevents back pain, it is not advisable to practice this posture if you are already suffering from back pain.

Sun Salutation (Surya Namaskar)

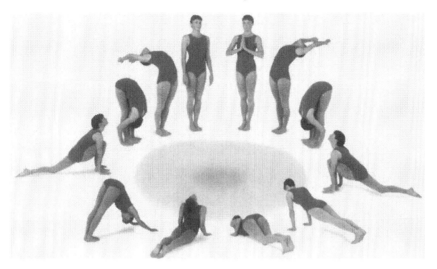

Surya Namaskar (Sun Salutation)

If you have practiced and mastered all the asanas described in this chapter, you are ready to take the next step. As we have to practice those postures sequentially, start sun salutation only if you have gained some degree of skill in the previous asanas. The asanas we are about to exercise are as follows.

1. *Pranamasana (Prayer pose)*

2. *Tadasana (Mountain pose)*

3. *Hasta Padasana (Hand to foot pose)*

4. *Aswa Sanchalanasana (Equestrian pose)--- Left foot*

5. *Dandasana (Stick pose)*

6. *Astangasana (Salute With eight parts Or points)*

7. *Bhujangasana (Cobra pose)*

8. *Adho-Mukha Svanasana (Downward-facing dog)*

9. *Aswa Sanchalanasana (Equestrian pose)--- Right foot*

10. *Hasta padasana (Hand to feet pose)--- Repetition*

11. *Tadasana (Mountain Pose)----- Repetition*

Now you have the list of postures, and we are going to practice back-to-back. As you have learnt all the asanas sun salutation will cover, there is no need for a detailed explanation of each pose here. We will rather learn how to maintain the sequence.

In the beginning, you will need to memorise the order of asanas in a sun salutation. Once the body gets used to the order, it will move spontaneously and switch from one pose to the next quite smoothly. Therefore you may find sun salutation a little hard in the beginning, in time you will do it with ease and start to enjoy. Sun salutation can be performed in different paces, like slow, medium and fast. And each pace has different sets of benefits. But to get the optimum benefit, we will do it slowly.

Stand at the edge of your mat with your feet slightly apart. Keep your body straight, shoulders relaxed. Breathe in, raise your hands and join the palms together in Pranamasana. Breathe in and out and feel the stress points. Stay in this position for five seconds. Then breathe in and lift your arms together above your head in Tadasana. Bend, your body, slightly back by pushing your pelvis forward. Stay for five seconds and be aware of the feelings in your joints and muscles. Breath-in. Breathe out and lower your hands to touch your feet. Switch your body to Hasta Padasana.

After five seconds, bring your hands to the floor. Move your left foot a few steps forward and position between the palms. Make sure that your knee is aligned with your ankle. Move the right foot a few steps back. You can bend the right knee to feel more comfortable. Breathe in and try to straighten your torso with the fingers touching the ground. Move your chin up and shift your gaze to the ceiling. This is Aswa Sanchalanasana. Stay for five seconds and breathe normally.

Exhale… step your left foot back to alignment with right foot. Lower your head and torso. You are now in Dandasana.

After five seconds breath out…bend your knees and elbows and rest your chest on the floor. Make sure your chin, palms, chest, knees, and toes are touching the ground. You are in Astanga Namaskara Position. Some experts advice to hold the breath in Astanga Namaskara, others recommend chanting the mantra.

Breathe in and lift your torso. Curve your spine back and raise your chin. Press the floor with your palms and try to straighten the hands. Bring your thighs in contact with the floor. Breathe out. You are in Bhujangasana.

Breathe normally and after five seconds, breathe out. Firm your legs and get your knees off the floor. Make sure your legs are straight, head lower and gaze fixed on the floor. You have switched to Adho-Mukha Svanasana. Now inhale and exhale naturally. Spend five seconds here.

Inhale and raise your torso. Push your right foot forward and place between the palms. Slightly step back your left foot and bend the knee. Curve your spine back and lift your chin up with your fingers touching the floor. This is Aswa Sanchalanasana again. But remember to use your right foot this time.

Once you are done, bring your left foot forward into alignment with your right foot. Keep your palms on the floor. Breathe in and straighten your legs. You are back in Hasta Padasana posture. If you find it difficult to keep your legs straight, you can bend your knees, but not too much. Remember to stay in this pose for five seconds.

Now breathe in, join your palms, raise your torso and move to the tadasana pose. Push your pelvis forward and bend backward. Once finished, stand in a relaxed posture with the hand by your sides.

This is just one round. Do more rounds. If you think that you are moving slowly, you can speed up the poses. Refrain yourself from putting too much pressure in any posture; it may cause injury. It is better to practice surya namaskar in the supervision of an expert. Practice surya namaskar at the beginning of yoga session. It is a good warm up yoga.

Benefits: You already know the benefits of each of the postures included in a sun salutation. But when all those Asanas come together in surya Namaskar, collectively they offer tremendous benefits. It is a very important set of postures in Yoga. Sun salutation counteracts aging, improves blood circulation, improves cardiac health, wards off stress and anxiety, elevates the mood, prevents diabetes and hypertension, boosts immunity, speeds up metabolism, gives you the perfect shape, improves vitality along with lots of other benefits.

Chapter 5

Boosting immunity

Yoga has enormous potentials to prevent physical and mental ailments. At any given moment there are above two hundred different viruses that can enter into our system. By eating balanced diets, having a proper sleep, and following few other healthy rules, we can cut the risks of common illnesses. But that is not enough. If we integrate yoga in our life, we will be more protected from most of the illnesses. Ancient masters of yoga believed that Yoga could prevent any disease. Most practitioners of modern day yoga claim that they feel a significant improvement in their physical immunity when they practice the asanas regularly. In this chapter, we will learn few postures that improve the functioning of some of our vital organs, and hence make our body immune to various sicknesses.

Shoulder Stand (Sarvangasana)

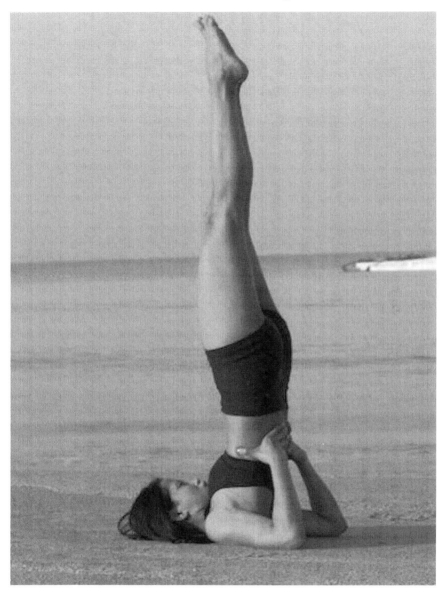

Sarvangasana (Shoulder Pose)

It is better to practice this asana against a wall to support the body until you feel balanced in this posture. Lie on your back. Take a couple of deep breaths. While exhaling, lift your legs and back with one movement. Keep your legs straight, and make sure that your shoulders are carrying the weight of your body. Support your back with your hands… place your palms on your lower back.

Now straighten your spine, but try not to press the neck into the floor. Your shoulders and upper arms are carrying your weight. Avoid putting pressure on your head and neck. If you find it difficult to stay steady, you can use the support wall to balance your body.

Join your feet together and fix your gaze on the big toes. Keep the legs straight. Now breathe naturally, and stay in this posture for 30 seconds to a minute. During this time, if you feel any strain in your neck, gently come out of this posture.

To descend from this pose, bend your knees and lower them to the forehead. Place your hands on the floor with palms facing down. Now slowly lower your torso without lifting your head. Bring your legs to the floor. Relax your body in savasana for a minute.

Benefits: Sarvangasana stabilizes the functions of thyroid and parathyroid glands by stimulating them. By practicing shoulder stand we can maintain a healthy gastrointestinal and enteric system, prevent dyspepsia and constipation. Regular practice promotes blood flow in the brain, so the brain cells get nourished with more blood. This posture stretches the heart muscles by causing more blood flow to the heart. On the top, this posture helps to immunise the body from various diseases.

Fish Pose (Matsyasana)

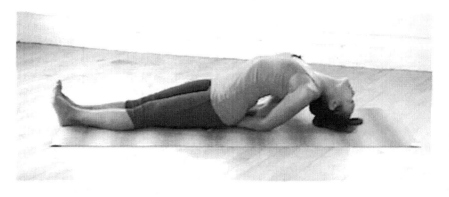

Matsyasana (Fish Pose)

In Sanskrit Matsya means fish. Therefore this pose resembles the position of a fish. In Astanga Vinyasa Yoga, the fish pose is considered as a counter pose of Sarvangasana. Therefore it is better to practice this asana after you are done with shoulder stand. There are variations in Fish pose. We will discuss the easiest one.

If you are resting in Savasana after practicing shoulder stand, bend your knees with your feet on the floor. Face your palms down. Exhale... slightly lift your pelvis and place your palms underneath your buttocks. Now your buttocks are resting on the back of your palms. Make sure both of your forearms are close to your torso.

Inhale and bend your spine towards the ceiling, press your shoulder blades on your back. Bend your elbow, and press your forearm and elbow against the floor. Allow your forearm and elbow to support your torso. Lift your head off the floor, then touch the floor with the tip of your head. Avoid putting much weight on your head. Let your elbows carry the weight of your upper body. Now straighten your legs and bring your heels on the floor. Join your big toes together. If you feel a strain in your neck, you can use a folded blanket underneath.

Breathe normally and stay in this position for thirty seconds to one minute.

Benefits: Matsyasana is called the destroyer of all diseases. This pose has therapeutic uses for curing constipation, respiratory illnesses, depression, backache, menstrual pain and so forth. Matsyasana normalizes the functions of pituitary, adrenaline, pineal and parathyroid glands. This pose is also good for the respiratory and digestive system.

Chapter 6

Releasing Stress and Anxiety

Most of the yoga postures have the potential for calming the anxious mind. But there are asans, which focus directly on relieving stress. Savasana (corpse pose) and Balasana (child pose), if performed correctly can bring a tranquil feeling. Advanced poses like Plough pose and Wheel pose are also effective for relieving stress.

In this chapter, we will discuss a posture called cow-cat pose for stress relief.

This posture is actually combined of two asasans. One is Cow pose (Bitilasana), and the other is Cat pose (Marjaryasana).

The Cow pose

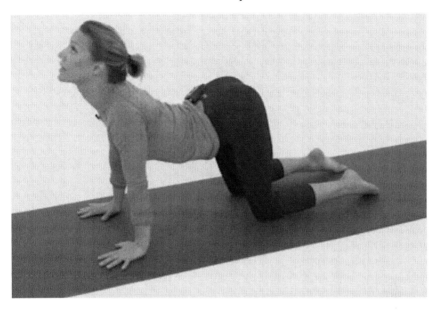

Bitilasana (Cow Pose)

Sit in vajrasana. With your knees and toes touching the ground, bring your thighs in a position perpendicular to the floor and place your palms on the floor. Knees apart, palms apart- fingers spread. So your hands and thighs are parallel to each other and perpendicular to the floor, in a 'table-top' position. Breathe in, lift your chin up and stretch your belly toward the floor. Chest up, gaze at the ceiling, keep inhaling. This is Cow pose (Bitilasana).

Now breathe out and lower your head and stretch you torso round up toward the ceiling, so that it looks like a cat stretching out. Keep exhaling. This is Cat pose (Marjaryasana)

Again breath in and lower your belly (cow-pose), breathe out and round-up your torso (cat pose).

Practice these two poses back and forth for a few more times.

Cow-Cat Pose is a good warm-up exercise. Therefore you can add this posture to your warm up session.

The Cat Pose

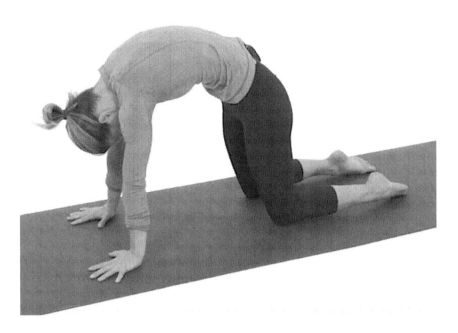

Marjaryasana (Cat Pose)

Cow-Cat pose is a posture for the absolute beginners and a perfect preparatory exercise before strenuous yoga postures. Apart from stress release, this exercise has other benefits including firming the back, chest, and belly, increasing the flexibility of the spine and maintaining overall physical and mental wellbeing. Benefits of cow-cat pose will be visible in few days of practice.

Headstand (Sirsasana)

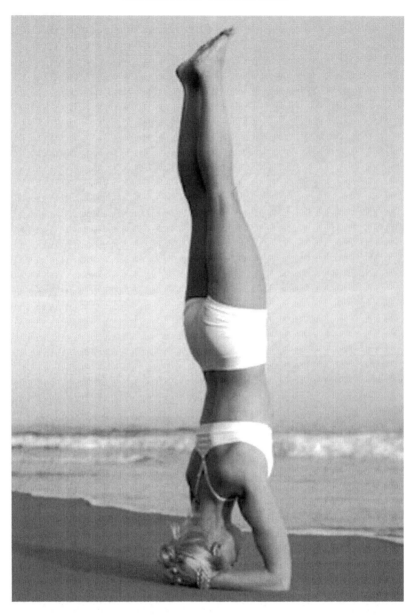

Shirsasana (HeadStand)

This posture may look scary, but it is not. You can master it in a day or two. Headstand is the most important pose among the inverted asanas. It is often termed as the king of all asanas. Traditionally this posture is practiced at the end of the yoga session. It is better to learn this asana in the presence of a qualified instructor. Don't try to learn this posture at the very first attempt. You have to be a little fearless, and take some caution in the beginning. Use the wall to support your body and to avoid injuries in the early days of practice.

Position yourself in Child pose. Bring your palms together and interlock your fingers. Place your head close to your wrists inside the triangle. Press your forearms and elbows and straighten your legs. Now your forearms, head, and feet are carrying your weight, and your position looks like inverted 'V'. Remember not to put much weight on your head. If you are practicing without an instructor, make sure somebody is present. Place your head almost a foot away from the wall when you are trying it for the first time.

Now breathe in and while breathing out, get your right foot off the ground first, and while straightening the right leg, push the ground with your left foot and get your left foot off the ground too. If you are using the support wall, use the wall to support your legs in the beginning. The best way to learn Shirsana is to get support from someone to help you to reach your legs to the wall. Both of your legs are now straight and joined together.

Let your forearms and elbows carry the most weight of your body. Put the minimum amount of weight on your head. Remember, you only need to practice this pose once to overcome the fear of falling. Once the fear is gone, you will find shirsasana to be the easiest of all postures. Breathe normally and stay for at least half a minute. You can stay in Shirsasana for up to five minutes.

To safely descend from this posture, bend your left knee and allow your left foot to reach the ground first. Bend the right knee and lower the right foot when the left foot is half way to the floor.

Benefits: Shirsana eliminates stress. It increases the blood flow in the head and reverses the sign of aging. This posture also calms the mind, promotes good sleep and reverses the effect of gravity in our organs.

Conclusion

To receive the long-term benefits of yoga, regularity is paramount. Even fifteen minutes of yoga practice will make a big difference. Remember to breathe and be mindful while you are doing the postures. Yoga is not only about the body; it is also about the mind. Therefore it is important to anchor the mind in the present during the practice. Do not try hard; your body may need some time to reach the desired level of flexibility. Be patient and stick to your practice. Don't push the body to the limit. Although it is a beginner's guide, most of the asanas should be suitable for anyone with normal health and average musculoskeletal flexibility. Still, if you don't feel confident enough to try any of those relatively advanced postures, get help from an instructor. Practice yoga every day, and you will be amazed by the transformation.

THE END

Stretch warm-up + cow-cat

① Sun salutation

② mountain → warrior 1 & 2 →
    Triangle → Tree

③ Shoulder → Plough → fish → wheel

④ Thunderbolt, child → headstand

⑤ Corpse

Notes

Made in the USA
Middletown, DE
26 April 2017